WHAT PEER EDUCATORS IN HIV EDUCATION AND PATIENTS SHOULD KNOW: WHAT PEER EDUCATORS IN HIV EDUCATION AND PATIENTS SHOULD KNOW

Dr. Kenneth Dantzler-Corbin

Copyright © 2020 Kenneth Dantzler-Corbin Name

All rights reserved.

ISBN: 9781658678551

DEDICATION

I dedicate this book to individuals who work with the HIV community and are living with HIV.

Table of Contents

Chapter 1 HIV is Manageable 6

    What researchers know about the single-tablet regimen 8

    What is the next phase after testing positive for HIV? 11

    The person may have questions about their HIV diagnosis 13

    History on HIV 17

    The Hunter Theory 21

Chapter 2 HIV Basics 27

    Knowing the Basics of HIV 27

    What is the definition of a virus? 27

    Life Cycle of HIV 31

    What is the link between the HIV life cycle and HIV medicines? 32

        Viral Attachment 34

        Viral Fusion 36

        The Encoding 37

        The Reverse Transcription 38

        Viral Latency 40

        Final Assembly 42

        Budding or Maturation 43

Chapter 3 Adherence to taking Medications 44

WHAT PEER EDUCATORS IN HIV EDUCATION AND PATIENTS SHOULD KNOW

Adherence 44
What is HIV treatment, adherence? 45
Interpersonal Relationship Role 47
Why is medication adherence significant to the patient? 48
Why did the patient forget to take the medication? ... 49
Asking questions concerning medications 50
Chapter 4 PreP as Prevention 52
Using PrEP as Prevention 52
Differences between prep and pep 54
Chapter 5 U=U 55
U=U in HIV care 55
What does suppression mean when talking about U=U? 56

Chapter 1 HIV is Manageable

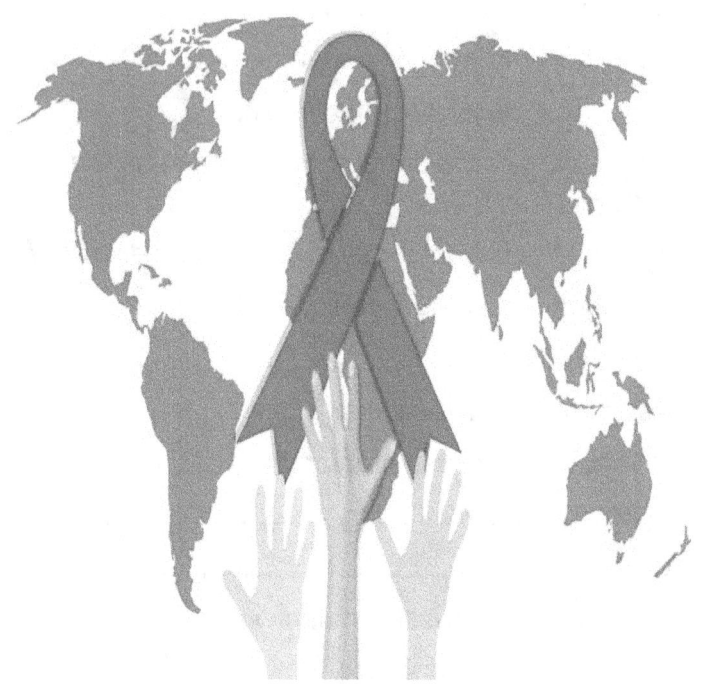

HIV is a manageable condition now than it was a few years ago. Three years following the first reports of HIV/AIDS published, a revolutionary analysis, carried out by the United States National Institutes of Health, noted that antiretroviral treatment plays a role in HIV prevention.[1] In discordant partners, where one partner had HIV, and the

---

[1] "HIV: from a devastating epidemic to a manageable - WHO." https://www.who.int/publications/10-year-review/hiv/en/. Accessed 25 Dec. 2019.

other didn't, remedy for the individuals with HIV led to a 96% reduction in transmission to the partner.[2]

The medications are better, with fewer side effects. An individual who has an HIV diagnosis does not mean that this individual is declining in health. Individuals can live a very active life and appreciate the years to come.

HIV patients on a single tablet daily regimen had better treatment retention and better suppression than patients taking multiple pills. HIV, or human immunodeficiency virus, weakens one's immune system.[3] It amplifies the risk of catching more frequent infections and conditions that do not affect people with a stronger immune system.[4] As the infection advances, it can lead to AIDS (Acquired Immunodeficiency Syndrome).[5]

---

[2] "HIV: from a devastating epidemic to a manageable - WHO." https://www.who.int/publications/10-year-review/hiv/en/. Accessed 25 Dec. 2019.

[3] "Single-tablet regimen for HIV: Benefits and drug chart." 10 Dec. 2018, https://www.medicalnewstoday.com/articles/323942.php. Accessed 27 Dec. 2019.

[4] "Single-Tablet Regimen for HIV: Benefits and More - Healthline." https://www.healthline.com/health/hiv-aids/single-tablet-regimen. Accessed 27 Dec. 2019.

[5] "Single-tablet regimens | aidsmap." 13 Jun. 2019, http://www.aidsmap.com/about-hiv/single-tablet-regimens. Accessed 27 Dec. 2019.

If untreated, the average survival time is 9 to 11 years.[6] The patient takes the newer treatment regimens once a day. Once-daily regimens are the new standards for HIV care.[7] Having to take medicine once a day decreases the pill burden, which could improve the patient's quality of life and treatment adherence.[8] The newest regimens require a single pill.

What researchers know about the single-tablet regimen

The single-tablet regimen makes progress. Researchers followed patients for a year and found that a single-tablet regimen compared favorably with the multiple tablet regimens.[9] Researchers measured three aspects of

---

[6] "Single-tablet regimen for HIV: Benefits and drug chart." 10 Dec. 2018, https://www.medicalnewstoday.com/articles/323942.php. Accessed 27 Dec. 2019.

[7] "Single-Tablet Regimen for HIV: Benefits and More - Healthline." https://www.healthline.com/health/hiv-aids/single-tablet-regimen. Accessed 27 Dec. 2019.

[8] "Single-Tablet Regimen for HIV: Benefits and More - Healthline." https://www.healthline.com/health/hiv-aids/single-tablet-regimen. Accessed 27 Dec. 2019.

[9] "HIV virologic response better with single-tablet once daily ...." 4 Dec. 2018, https://www.ncbi.nlm.nih.gov/pmc/articles/PMC6295695/. Accessed 27 Dec. 2019.

WHAT PEER EDUCATORS IN HIV EDUCATION AND PATIENTS SHOULD KNOW

treatment: adherence, retention, and HIV suppression.[10]

Patients are more adherent to a single-tablet regimen. HIV adherence means that the patient took their medications over 80% of the time, based on the prescriptions field.[11] The two regiments' rates of adherence were similar.[12], [13]

Patients in care have healthier success. To show the retention of patients in care, the patient had to visit the medical professional at two times, at least three months apart, during the first year for viral load measurements.[14] 81% of the single-tablet group showed retention,

---

[10] "HIV virologic response better with single-tablet once daily ...." 4 Dec. 2018, https://www.ncbi.nlm.nih.gov/pmc/articles/PMC6295695/. Accessed 27 Dec. 2019.

[11] "Single-tablet regimens | aidsmap." 13 Jun. 2019, http://www.aidsmap.com/about-hiv/single-tablet-regimens. Accessed 27 Dec. 2019.

[12] "Single-tablet regimens | aidsmap." 13 Jun. 2019, http://www.aidsmap.com/about-hiv/single-tablet-regimens. Accessed 27 Dec. 2019.

[13] "Single-tablet regimens | aidsmap." 13 Jun. 2019, http://www.aidsmap.com/about-hiv/single-tablet-regimens. Accessed 27 Dec. 2019.

[14] "Single-tablet regimens | aidsmap." 13 Jun. 2019, http://www.aidsmap.com/about-hiv/single-tablet-regimens. Accessed 27 Dec. 2019.

compared with 73% of the multiple-tablet groups.[15]

HIV suppression is the goal to reach when talking about adherence. HIV suppression measures the viral load in the blood of fewer than 400 copies per milliliter.[16] A single-tablet group suppresses 84% of the virus in the first year. In the multi tablet group, 78 percent showed suppression.[17]

If one has not been learning about the latest HIV medications, having a definite diagnosis can upset the person. New drugs are coming out each year, and people are living longer. One may know a little about HIV or AIDS, or perhaps one may know someone with this disease. The aim is to make sure that everyone has adequate information about this disease.

---

[15] "Single-tablet regimens | aidsmap." 13 Jun. 2019, http://www.aidsmap.com/about-hiv/single-tablet-regimens. Accessed 27 Dec. 2019.

[16] "Single-tablet regimens | aidsmap." 13 Jun. 2019, http://www.aidsmap.com/about-hiv/single-tablet-regimens. Accessed 27 Dec. 2019.

[17] "Single-tablet regimens | aidsmap." 13 Jun. 2019, http://www.aidsmap.com/about-hiv/single-tablet-regimens. Accessed 27 Dec. 2019.

What is the next phase after testing positive for HIV?

If one has had sexual contact with any person, have an HIV test by a professional. Testing for HIV for the first time can be challenging. Testing positive for HIV leaves an individual with questions and issues. It is important to remember that HIV is a manageable disease addressed with HIV medicines.[18]

The first step after testing positive would be to see a health care provider, even if the person does not feel ill. HIV+ person works with their health care providers. The patient and the doctor decide when to begin HIV medications and what HIV medicines to take.[19]

The usage of HIV medicines to deal with HIV illness is known as antiretroviral treatment (ART).[20] Individuals on

---

[18] "Just Diagnosed: Next Steps After Testing Positive for HIV ...." 18 Jan. 2019, https://aidsinfo.nih.gov/understanding-hiv-aids/fact-sheets/21/65/just-diagnosed--next-steps-after-testing-positive-for-hiv. Accessed 25 Dec. 2019.

[19] "Just Diagnosed: Next Steps After Testing Positive for HIV ...." 18 Jan. 2019, https://aidsinfo.nih.gov/understanding-hiv-aids/fact-sheets/21/65/just-diagnosed--next-steps-after-testing-positive-for-hiv. Accessed 25 Dec. 2019.

[20] "HIV Medications: Combinations, Antiretrovirals, HAART, & More." 20 Oct. 2019, https://www.webmd.com/hiv-aids/hiv-medications. Accessed 27 Dec. 2019.

ART take a combination of HIV medicines (called an HIV treatment regimen) every day.[21] ART stops HIV from spreading and reduces the quantity of HIV in the body. ART cannot cure HIV.[22] It assists people with HIV to live longer, healthier lifestyles and lessens the risk of HIV transmission.[23]

People with HIV should begin ART. In people with HIV who have conditions, such as specific HIV-related ailments and confections, it is essential to start ART immediately.[24] Deciding when one should start ART and what HIV medicines to take has an HIV standard evaluation.[25]

---

[21] "HIV: Antiretroviral Therapy (ART) - Types, Brand Names, How ...." 22 Oct. 2019, https://www.webmd.com/hiv-aids/aids-hiv-medication. Accessed 27 Dec. 2019.

[22] "HIV: Antiretroviral Therapy (ART) - Types, Brand Names, How ...." 22 Oct. 2019, https://www.webmd.com/hiv-aids/aids-hiv-medication. Accessed 27 Dec. 2019.

[23] "HIV Medications: NRTIs, Protease Inhibitors, and Much More." https://www.healthline.com/health/hiv-aids/medications-list. Accessed 27 Dec. 2019.

[24] "HIV Medicines and Side Effects | Understanding HIV/AIDS ...." 24 Oct. 2019, https://aidsinfo.nih.gov/understanding-hiv-aids/fact-sheets/22/63/hiv-medicines-and-side-effects. Accessed 27 Dec. 2019.

[25] "Just Diagnosed: Next Steps After Testing Positive for HIV ...." 18 Jan. 2019, https://aidsinfo.nih.gov/understanding-hiv-aids/fact-sheets/21/65/just-diagnosed--next-steps-after-testing-positive-for-

WHAT PEER EDUCATORS IN HIV EDUCATION AND PATIENTS SHOULD KNOW

The person may have questions about their HIV diagnosis

People detected HIV infection could have many concerns. If one has tested HIV positive, one may have a few of the questions:

- Because the individual has HIV, will the individual get AIDS?
- So, what can the individual do to remain healthy and steer free of getting other viruses?
- How does the person prevent passing HIV to another person?
- How will HIV treatment affect the individual's life?
- How should the individual communicate with their companion that the person has HIV?
- Should the individual tell their employer or the ones the person work with that they have HIV?
- Are there support groups for persons with HIV?
- Are there any resources offered to help the person purchase their HIV medications?

Lots of people find it useful to write concerns before a medical visit. These individuals need to bring a relative or buddy to their HIV appointments. The individuals help to

---

hiv. Accessed 25 Dec. 2019.

remind the patient of questions he or she may ask the provider.[26]

When getting a result, individuals reply in different situations. Whatever one believes about the virus, the person needs to be in care. People living with HIV can have a full life and live an average life expectancy the key is coming to one's doctor's appointment and taking one's medications as prescribed by a medical specialist. [27]

The misinformation and myths we hear many times. It would be best if one remembered that having HIV means many things. For example, a person having HIV does not mean that that individual has AIDS. An HIV positive test result means that one may have the virus. Having HIV does not mean that one will feel the effects of the virus, nor does it mean that this individual may have aids.

Sometimes, the individual may not be HIV medication for many years. Depending on how their immune system response to the virus, the way to be sure is to talk with one's medical provider and ask questions about one's HIV test results. The person's blood can tell one how strong

---

[26] "10 Things Everyone Should Understand About HIV And AIDS ...." 28 Oct. 2016, https://www.self.com/story/facts-about-hiv-and-aids. Accessed 25 Dec. 2019.

[27] "Living with HIV: What is it really like? - Medical News Today." 13 Dec. 2018,
https://www.medicalnewstoday.com/articles/323981.php.
Accessed 25 Dec. 2019.

one's immune system may be.

The new HIV medications coming out are getting better each year. The good news is that HIV is not just about medicine, which is effective and safe when the patient uses the medication. Years ago, doctors made many decisions on how researchers would fight the virus and which drugs used in the patient.

Sometimes, the doctors prescribed a combination of medications, and now there is one pill a day with a combination of many medicines in one pill. Today, individuals take a single, once-a-day, fixed-dose tablet that combines many medications. It is much simpler to manage and has fewer unwanted effects.[28]

The standard of care to suppress the virus is for the patient to begin treatment after diagnosis and continue to take medication for the rest of their life.[29]

This strategy revolutionized how we consider HIV avoidance. Five years ago, we learned that the moment

---

[28] "How HIV became a treatable, chronic disease." 2 Dec. 2015, http://theconversation.com/how-hiv-became-a-treatable-chronic-disease-51238. Accessed 25 Dec. 2019.

[29] "How HIV became a treatable, chronic disease." 2 Dec. 2015, http://theconversation.com/how-hiv-became-a-treatable-chronic-disease-51238. Accessed 25 Dec. 2019.

clients take these medicines and suppress HIV replication, they are much less prone to transmit HIV to another person.[30]

In 2012, the U.S. Foods and Drug Administration approved the medication that first protects those who do not have HIV from infection, termed pre-exposure prophylaxis (PrEP). Today, the Centers for infection Control and Prevention (CDC) and the World Health Organization endorse PrEP, in grouping with behavioral interventions, for people at high risk of getting HIV, for instance, men who have sexual intercourse with men and couples where one partner is HIV-infected.

A person can go on to have an active and full life. An individual can become very productive in whatever field of study or pursue a career that means a career in medicine. HIV should not stop the person from pursuing their life girl. There are no medical reasons. One cannot just be as active as one was before.

---

[30] "How HIV became a treatable, chronic disease." 2 Dec. 2015, http://theconversation.com/how-hiv-became-a-treatable-chronic-disease-51238. **Accessed 25 Dec. 2019.**

WHAT PEER EDUCATORS IN HIV EDUCATION AND PATIENTS SHOULD KNOW

History on HIV

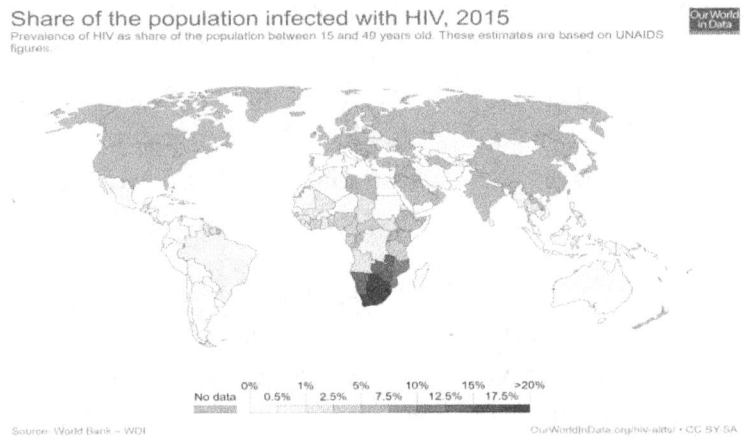

The history of HIV and the AIDS epidemic began in illness, fear, and death as the World's face is a new and unknown virus.[31] Some believed that HIV originated in Kinshasa, in the Democratic Republic of Congo around 1920 with HIV crossed species from chimpanzees to humans.[32] Until the 1980s, scientists had no number of infected people with HIV.[33]

---

[31] "History of HIV and AIDS overview | Avert."
https://www.avert.org/professionals/history-hiv-aids/overview.
Accessed 27 Dec. 2019.

[32] "History of HIV and AIDS overview | Avert."
https://www.avert.org/professionals/history-hiv-aids/overview.
Accessed 27 Dec. 2019.

[33] "History of HIV and AIDS overview | Avert."
https://www.avert.org/professionals/history-hiv-aids/overview.

HIV was unknown, and in transmission, one did not see noticeable signs or symptoms. Experts documented sporadic cases of aids. The experts had available data of the current epidemic in the mid to late 1970s by 1980; HIV spread to five continents North America, South America, Europe, Africa, and Australia.[34] HIV infected 100,000 and 300 people.[35]

The HIV/AIDS epidemic began in the year 1981 became an intense subject.[36] The HIV epidemic has produced many theories. One theory is that the polio vaccine went bad; another theory was that it was secret germ warfare that the government was performing on human beings.[37] The earliest HIV epidemic evidence was between 1910 and 1930. Researchers and scientists know that there was a spread of HIV throughout Africa for 70 years before

---

Accessed 27 Dec. 2019.

[34] "History of HIV and AIDS overview | Avert." https://www.avert.org/professionals/history-hiv-aids/overview. Accessed 27 Dec. 2019.

[35] "History of HIV and AIDS overview | Avert." https://www.avert.org/professionals/history-hiv-aids/overview. Accessed 27 Dec. 2019.

[36] "History of HIV and AIDS overview | Avert." https://www.avert.org/professionals/history-hiv-aids/overview. Accessed 27 Dec. 2019.

[37] "AIDS Timeline." http://www.factlv.org/timeline.htm. Accessed 27 Dec. 2019.

discovered.[38] Since the time of its discovery, HIV has undergone small genetic changes creating subtypes of HIV.[39]

Scientists and researchers traced the spread of the subtype of HIV geographically. Scientists can trace the predominant strain of HIV in the United States and to Africa. Researchers around the World looked for the origin of HIV soon after they determined this disease caused AIDS. These researchers discovered a close cousin to HIV in monkeys and chimpanzees. Experts called the virus SIV or simian immunodeficiency virus. An HIV-like virus that inflected monkeys and apes and caused illness, much like AIDS. [40]

SIV cannot infect humans, and HIV cannot infect monkeys.[41] Though, scientists did a study on the blood of

---

[38] "A Timeline of HIV and AIDS | HIV.gov." https://www.hiv.gov/hiv-basics/overview/history/hiv-and-aids-timeline. Accessed 27 Dec. 2019.

[39] "Thirty Years of HIV/AIDS: Snapshots of an Epidemic - amfAR." https://www.amfar.org/thirty-years-of-hiv/aids-snapshots-of-an-epidemic/. Accessed 27 Dec. 2019.

[40] "Simian Immunodeficiency Virus (SIV) | Definition | AIDSinfo." https://aidsinfo.nih.gov/understanding-hiv-aids/glossary/660/simian-immunodeficiency-virus. Accessed 25 Dec. 2019.

[41] "Simian Immunodeficiency Virus (SIV) | Definition | AIDSinfo." https://aidsinfo.nih.gov/understanding-hiv-aids/glossary/660/simian-immunodeficiency-virus. Accessed 25 Dec.

a woman and found her HIV to be a unique variant having characteristics of both HIV and SIV. Some scientists suggest that SIV somehow changed over time and became HIV.

Recognition of the primate source that spawned the HIV-1 pandemic is of scientific and public health importance. It is now well-known that the immediate precursor of HIV-1 is a lentivirus that infects chimpanzees of the subspecies Pan troglodytes in west-central Africa. What is understood but perhaps less commonly valued is that SIVcpz strains transmitted to individuals on at least three individual occurrences and that the present HIV-1 group M pandemic, which has stricken over 60 million people and caused over 20 million fatalities, lead from one of these transmission occasions in the 1st half of the 20th century? The reason for HIV-1's sudden emergence, the adaptive changes that followed, and the mechanisms underlying its pathogenicity that is unique though not yet determined.[42]

Primates naturally infected with SIV, including chimpanzees that are SIVcpz-infected, appear not to develop immunodeficiency or AIDS. In contrast, some view the HIV illness of humans as a recent loss of CD4+ T lymphocytes, chronic immune activation, and the

---

2019.

[42] "Simian Immunodeficiency Virus Infection of Chimpanzees ...." https://jvi.asm.org/content/79/7/3891. Accessed 25 Dec. 2019.

gradual destruction of an array of resistant functions. The scientists did not understand the foundation in pathogenicity. These experts deciphered the viral and/or host factors accountable for the nonpathogenic Nature of SIV infections. This discovery was beneficial in developing a more effective treatment for HIV/AIDS.[43]

Genomes of chimps and humans are similar. Chimpanzees and human beings have 98% of characteristics across their genomes.[44] This level of relatedness supplies an opportunity that is a unique search for critical differences in virus-host interactions accountable for changes in viral pathogenicity. This approach could show complementary to present studies that focus on human illness susceptibility.[45]

The Hunter Theory

The Hunter Theory was part of the HIV/AIDS understanding of the early stages of the disease. Scientists recognized Acquired Immune Deficiency Syndrome or AIDS as a new infection or disease in 1981 when

---

[43] "Simian Immunodeficiency Virus - an overview | ScienceDirect ...." https://www.sciencedirect.com/topics/medicine-and-dentistry/simian-immunodeficiency-virus. Accessed 25 Dec. 2019.

[44] "Simian Immunodeficiency Virus Infection of Chimpanzees ...." https://jvi.asm.org/content/79/7/3891. Accessed 25 Dec. 2019.

[45] "Simian Immunodeficiency Virus Infection of Chimpanzees ...." https://jvi.asm.org/content/79/7/3891. Accessed 25 Dec. 2019.

increasing numbers of young gay men succumbed to uncommon opportunistic infections and rare malignancies.[46] Scientists noted that a retrovirus classified as human immunodeficiency virus type 1 (HIV-1), as the causative cause of what has since become one of the most devastating infectious diseases that developed in recent history.[47]

Researchers looked for ways to understand how individuals got infected with HIV. HIV-1 spreads by sexual intercourse, percutaneous, and perinatal routes; 80% of men and women receive HIV-1 subsequent exposure at mucosal surfaces, and AIDS is a sexually transmitted disease.[48] Since its first identification of the disease almost three decades ago, the widespread form of HIV-1, also called the leading (M) group, has infected at least 60 million people and prompted over 25 million

---

[46] "Origins of HIV and the AIDS Pandemic - NCBI." https://www.ncbi.nlm.nih.gov/pmc/articles/PMC3234451/. Accessed 26 Dec. 2019.

[47] "Origins of HIV and the AIDS Pandemic - NCBI." https://www.ncbi.nlm.nih.gov/pmc/articles/PMC3234451/. Accessed 26 Dec. 2019.

[48] "Origins of HIV and the AIDS Pandemic - NCBI." https://www.ncbi.nlm.nih.gov/pmc/articles/PMC3234451/. Accessed 26 Dec. 2019.

death cases.[49]

Countries experienced many deaths because of HIV/AIDS. Developing countries have experienced the most significant HIV/AIDS morbidity and death rate, with the highest prevalence rates reported in adolescent men and women in sub-Saharan Africa.[50] Though antiretroviral treatment reduced the toll of AIDS-related deaths, admittance to therapy was not characteristic, and the predictions of curative treatments and an effective vaccine were uncertain. [51]For that reason, AIDS continued to present a public health threat for many years.[52] **This theory pointed toward African tribes. Within the lack of direct proof, a thought "cut hunter" appears in the index patient of pandemic HIV/AIDS.[53]**

---

[49] "Origins of HIV and the AIDS Pandemic - NCBI."
https://www.ncbi.nlm.nih.gov/pmc/articles/PMC3234451/.
Accessed 26 Dec. 2019.

[50] "Opportunistic Infections and AIDS-Related Cancers - HIV InSite."
14 Sep. 2011, http://hivinsite.ucsf.edu/insite?page=pb-diag-04-00.
Accessed 26 Dec. 2019.

[51] "Origins of HIV and the AIDS Pandemic - NCBI."
https://www.ncbi.nlm.nih.gov/pmc/articles/PMC3234451/.
Accessed 26 Dec. 2019.

[52] "Origins of HIV and the AIDS Pandemic - NCBI."
https://www.ncbi.nlm.nih.gov/pmc/articles/PMC3234451/.
Accessed 26 Dec. 2019.

[53] "Beyond the Cut Hunter: A Historical Epidemiology of HIV ...."

WHAT PEER EDUCATORS IN HIV EDUCATION AND PATIENTS SHOULD KNOW

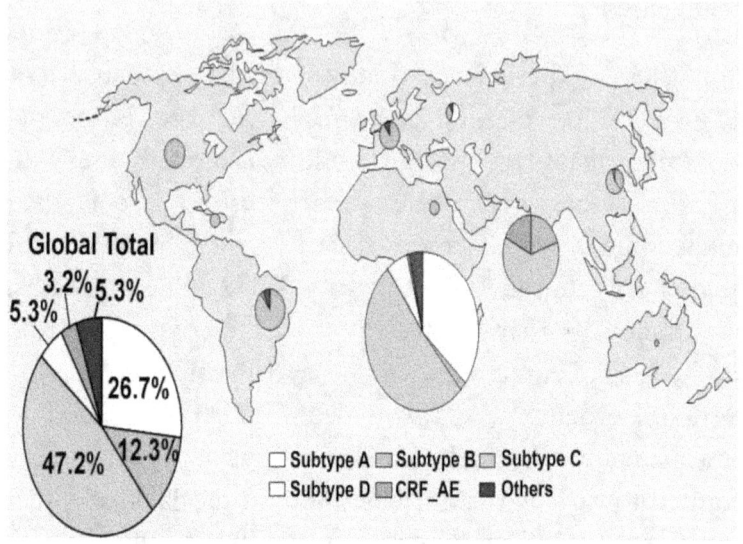

A hunter received a cut or injury from searching or butchering chimpanzees contaminated with simian immunodeficiency virus, causing the very first suffered human infection with the virus that could emerge as HIV-1M.[54] The "cut hunter" used a historical misunderstanding and ecological oversimplification of human-chimpanzee (Pan Troglodytes troglodytes) interactions that facilitated pathogenic transmission.[55]

---

https://www.ncbi.nlm.nih.gov/pubmed/27718030. Accessed 25 Dec. 2019.

[54] "Beyond the Cut Hunter: A Historical Epidemiology of HIV ...." https://www.ncbi.nlm.nih.gov/pubmed/27718030. Accessed 25 Dec. 2019.

[55] "Beyond the Cut Hunter: A Historical Epidemiology of HIV ...." https://www.ncbi.nlm.nih.gov/pubmed/27718030. Accessed 25

The reason scientists looked at this theory was that there was an extensive amount of monkey meat in some diet of individuals who lived in Africa. Experts theorized that individuals eating infected monkey meat caused the infection, exposing them to the virus — the SIV subtype.[56]

The question is, did HIV come from monkeys? In 1999, researchers found a strand of SIV in many of the monkeys they were studying, such as chimpanzees. Chimpanzees are identical to human beings.

The researchers discovered disconnection concluded that improve the chimpanzees was the source of HIV-1. The virus had to have some points across species from chimpanzees to human beings. Some scientists conducted more research on SIV to see how this virus developed. A scientist explored the hunter theory; they looked at the transmission of the virus from animals to human beings.[57]

Researchers found that individuals killed and ate these animals. The blood got into a wound on the people while

---

Dec. 2019.

[56] "Origin of HIV & AIDS | Avert."
https://www.avert.org/professionals/history-hiv-aids/origin.
Accessed 25 Dec. 2019.

[57] "Origin of HIV & AIDS | Avert."
https://www.avert.org/professionals/history-hiv-aids/origin.
Accessed 25 Dec. 2019.

hunting, and this was the way the virus transmitted from chimp to human beings. [58]

---

[58] "'Man the Hunter' theory is debunked in new book | The Source ...." 18 Feb. 2006, https://source.wustl.edu/2006/02/man-the-hunter-theory-is-debunked-in-new-book/. Accessed 25 Dec. 2019.

Chapter 2 HIV Basics

Knowing the Basics of HIV

To understand HIV and AIDS, the person needs a good understanding and knowledge and understanding of HIV. The individual must build a sound foundation if they want to live a productive life with HIV. To build a successful life and be healthy is to learn that all the patients can learn about HIV.

What is the definition of a virus?

This virus is a microscopic living organism that makes copies by using genetic materials from a living host. The virus is a small organism that cannot replicate on its own.[59]

This virus is small but has intelligence. When it infects a susceptible host, a virus can direct the cellular machinery to produce more viruses.[60] Many viruses have either RNA or DNA as genetic material.[61] The nucleic acid is a single-

---

[59] "Viruses: Structure, Function, and Uses - Molecular Cell ...." https://www.ncbi.nlm.nih.gov/books/NBK21523/. Accessed 25 Dec. 2019.

[60] "Viruses: Structure, Function, and Uses - Molecular Cell ...." https://www.ncbi.nlm.nih.gov/books/NBK21523/. Accessed 25 Dec. 2019.

[61] "Viruses: Structure, Function, and Uses - Molecular Cell ...." https://www.ncbi.nlm.nih.gov/books/NBK21523/. Accessed 25 Dec. 2019.

or double-stranded.[62] The infectious virus particle makes what we call a viron. The viron comprises the nucleic acid and an outer part of the protein.[63] The simplest viruses have just enough RNA or DNA to encode four proteins. The most complex encodes 100—200 proteins.[64]

HIV needs a host to live inside. HIV is in the genetic material, and that uses the genetic material to make a new HIV.[65] There are two genetic materials that the virus needs to make copies of RNA ribonucleic acid and DNA deoxyribonucleic acid.[66]

Scientists and researchers believed the human body comprises many substances and compounds that work

---

[62] "Viruses: Structure, Function, and Uses - Molecular Cell ...." https://www.ncbi.nlm.nih.gov/books/NBK21523/. Accessed 25 Dec. 2019.

[63] "Viruses: Structure, Function, and Uses - Molecular Cell ...." https://www.ncbi.nlm.nih.gov/books/NBK21523/. Accessed 25 Dec. 2019.

[64] "Viruses: Structure, Function, and Uses - Molecular Cell ...." https://www.ncbi.nlm.nih.gov/books/NBK21523/. Accessed 25 Dec. 2019.

[65] "How HIV Infects a Cell | International Partnership For ...." https://www.ipmglobal.org/how-hiv-infects-cell. Accessed 27 Dec. 2019.

[66] "What Are Viruses? | Live Science." 6 Jan. 2016, https://www.livescience.com/53272-what-is-a-virus.html. Accessed 25 Dec. 2019.

together to make us who we are. What is the substance's protein? In the human body, proteins are the building blocks. Proteins come together to form tissues, muscles, and organs.[67]

The DNA is a double strand of protein that comprises genetic material or information needed to manufacture new proteins.[68] The RNA is a single strand protein that transports DNA and controls the synthesis of new proteins. This genetic information makes a virus a virus.[69] There is a chemical reaction that goes on in the cell world; DNA changed to RNA inside the human body.[70]

The RNA transports the genetic code of the DNA to the site of the protein manufacturing.[71] This stage sounds as if

---

[67] "Viral Infection | Viral Infection Symptoms | MedlinePlus." https://medlineplus.gov/viralinfections.html. Accessed 25 Dec. 2019.

[68] "What is DNA? - Genetics Home Reference - NIH." 10 Dec. 2019, https://ghr.nlm.nih.gov/primer/basics/dna. Accessed 25 Dec. 2019.

[69] "DNA (Deoxyribonucleic Acid) | Talking Glossary of Genetic ...." https://www.genome.gov/genetics-glossary/Deoxyribonucleic-Acid. Accessed 25 Dec. 2019.

[70] "DNA (Deoxyribonucleic Acid) | Talking Glossary of Genetic ...." https://www.genome.gov/genetics-glossary/Deoxyribonucleic-Acid. Accessed 25 Dec. 2019.

[71] "RNA transport - Latest research and news | Nature." https://www.nature.com/subjects/rna-transport. Accessed 25 Dec. 2019.

there is an assembly going on inside the cell.[72] The RNA brings the genetic parts to the protein assembly line inside the cell.[73]

DNA inside the cell converts to RNA to replicate or make copies. HIV is a retrovirus. DNA inside the cell converts to RNA to replicate or make copies. HIV is what one may call a retrovirus. [74]This conversion means that there is a conversion process that takes place RNA to DNA. In this process, the retrovirus needs genetic material from a living host to multiply or survive.[75]

---

[72] "RNA transport - Latest research and news | Nature." https://www.nature.com/subjects/rna-transport. Accessed 25 Dec. 2019.

[73] "RNA transport - Latest research and news | Nature." https://www.nature.com/subjects/rna-transport. Accessed 25 Dec. 2019.

[74] "RNA Transport and Local Control of Translation - NCBI." https://www.ncbi.nlm.nih.gov/pmc/articles/PMC1850961/. Accessed 25 Dec. 2019.

[75] "RNA Transport and Local Control of Translation - NCBI." https://www.ncbi.nlm.nih.gov/pmc/articles/PMC1850961/. Accessed 25 Dec. 2019.

WHAT PEER EDUCATORS IN HIV EDUCATION AND PATIENTS SHOULD KNOW

Life Cycle of HIV

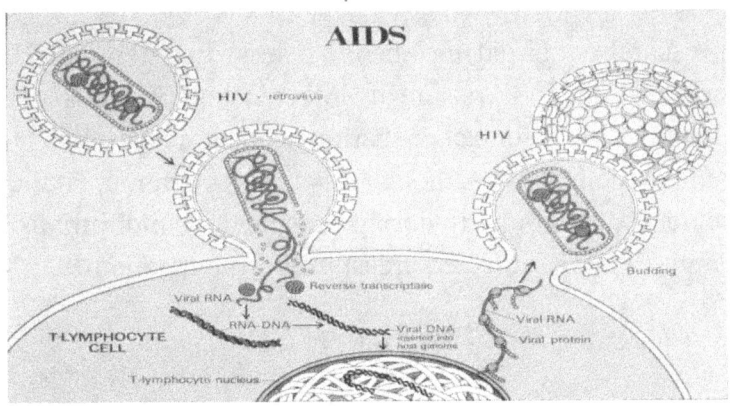

(https://commons.wikimedia.org/wiki/File:AIDS_life_cycle_illustration.jpg)

The life-cycle of HIV has several physiologic steps. HIV strikes and destroys the CD4 cells considering the immunity.[76] CD4 cells or white blood cell that plays a significant part in protecting the body from infection.

HIV uses the machinery of the CD4 cells to multiply and expand through the entire body.[77] This progression carried out in seven steps or stages of the HIV life cycle.[78] Each

---

[76] "Dissecting How CD4 T Cells Are Lost During HIV Infection." https://www.ncbi.nlm.nih.gov/pmc/articles/PMC4835240/. Accessed 26 Dec. 2019.

[77] "The HIV Life Cycle | Understanding HIV/AIDS | AIDSinfo." 1 Jul. 2019, https://aidsinfo.nih.gov/understanding-hiv-aids/fact-sheets/19/73/the-hiv-life-cycle. Accessed 26 Dec. 2019.

[78] "How HIV Destroys Immune Cells, Blocking HIV Cell Death ...." 18

step has a specific role in the replication of HIV.[79]

Researchers based the theory behind the steps on HIV medications.[80] Exposure to infected bodily fluids while having sexual contact or sharing needles are ways the HIV enters the body.[81] Although this is less common, HIV can enter a person's body during pregnancy, childbirth, or by ingesting HIV infected breast milk from the mother.[82]

What is the link between the HIV life cycle and HIV medicines?

Antiretroviral therapy (ART) is the utilization of HIV medicines to treat HIV infection. Persons on ART take a combination of HIV medicines (called an HIV regimen)

Dec. 2013, http://www.natap.org/2013/HIV/122713_02.htm. Accessed 26 Dec. 2019.

[79] "The HIV Life Cycle | Understanding HIV/AIDS | AIDSinfo." 1 Jul. 2019, https://aidsinfo.nih.gov/understanding-hiv-aids/fact-sheets/19/73/the-hiv-life-cycle. Accessed 25 Dec. 2019.

[80] "Antiretroviral Therapy for HIV Infection: Overview, FDA ...." 18 Apr. 2019, https://emedicine.medscape.com/article/1533218-overview. Accessed 25 Dec. 2019.

[81] "Life Cycle | Definition | AIDSinfo." https://aidsinfo.nih.gov/understanding-hiv-aids/glossary/1596/life-cycle. Accessed 25 Dec. 2019.

[82] "The HIV Life Cycle | Understanding HIV/AIDS | AIDSinfo." 1 Jul. 2019, https://aidsinfo.nih.gov/understanding-hiv-aids/fact-sheets/19/73/the-hiv-life-cycle. Accessed 25 Dec. 2019.

every day.[83] HIV medicines safeguard the immune system by blocking HIV at different stages of the HIV life cycle.[84]

Researchers based the HIV medication on the stages of HIV. Researchers categorized HIV medicines into diverse drug classes based on how they fight HIV.[85] The scientist designed each variety of drugs to target a step in the HIV life cycle.[86] Because HIV treatment comprises HIV medicines from at least two different HIV drug classes, ART helps to prevent HIV from multiplying.[87]

---

[83] "ART access-related barriers faced by HIV-positive persons ...." 7 Dec. 2016, https://www.ncbi.nlm.nih.gov/pmc/articles/PMC5142337/. Accessed 27 Dec. 2019.

[84] "ART access-related barriers faced by HIV-positive persons ...." 7 Dec. 2016, https://www.ncbi.nlm.nih.gov/pmc/articles/PMC5142337/. Accessed 27 Dec. 2019.

[85] "HIV Medications: NRTIs, Protease Inhibitors, and Much More." https://www.healthline.com/health/hiv-aids/medications-list. Accessed 27 Dec. 2019.

[86] "Management of HIV/AIDS - Wikipedia." https://en.wikipedia.org/wiki/Management_of_HIV/AIDS. Accessed 27 Dec. 2019.

[87] "Here's Why the First Cure for HIV Could Emerge from ...." 5 Nov. 2019, https://biobuzz.io/heres-why-the-first-cure-for-hiv-could-emerge-from-maryland/. Accessed 27 Dec. 2019.

Having less HIV in the human body protects the immune system and prevents HIV from advancing to AIDS. ART cannot cure HIV, but HIV medicines help people with HIV live longer, healthier lives. HIV medicines decrease the risk of HIV transmission (the spread of HIV to others).

Viral Attachment

Once HIV is in the body, this virus needs a host to attach itself to make copies. Specific virus attachment to entry receptors leads to productive routes in the host cells.[88] The host, in this case, is a specialized cell from the immune system. These cells are T cells or CD4 cells. CD4 cells or white blood cells play a critical role within the immune system.[89]

CD4 cells are the fighter cells. The CD4 cell count shows the health of one's immune system—the body's defense natural against pathogens, infections, and ailments.[90] CD4 cells are sometimes also referred to as T-cells, T-

---

[88] "Virus Attachment - an overview | ScienceDirect Topics." https://www.sciencedirect.com/topics/medicine-and-dentistry/virus-attachment. Accessed 25 Dec. 2019.

[89] "CD4 cell counts | aidsmap." 31 May. 2017, https://www.aidsmap.com/about-hiv/cd4-cell-counts. Accessed 25 Dec. 2019.

[90] "CD4 cell counts | aidsmap." 31 May. 2017, https://www.aidsmap.com/about-hiv/cd4-cell-counts. Accessed 25 Dec. 2019.

lymphocytes, or helper cells.[91]

The CD4 cell count is the number of bloodstream cells in a cubic millimeter of blood (a small blood sample). It is not a total count of all the CD4 cells in the body.[92] A higher quantity shows a more robust immune system.[93] Though, many times individuals referred to these cells as helper cells[94]. The CD4 cells fight against HIV. Once HIV is in the bloodstream, IV attaches itself to the CD4 cells.[95]

---

[91] "CD4 cell counts | aidsmap." 31 May. 2017, https://www.aidsmap.com/about-hiv/cd4-cell-counts. Accessed 25 Dec. 2019.

[92] "CD4 cell counts | aidsmap." 31 May. 2017, https://www.aidsmap.com/about-hiv/cd4-cell-counts. Accessed 25 Dec. 2019.

[93] "CD4 Count, HIV, and AIDS: Test and Results, What They Mean." 23 Jun. 2019, https://www.webmd.com/hiv-aids/cd4-count-what-does-it-mean. Accessed 25 Dec. 2019.

[94] "Viral attachment to host cell - UniProt." https://www.uniprot.org/keywords/KW-1161. Accessed 25 Dec. 2019.

[95] "Viral attachment to host cell - UniProt." https://www.uniprot.org/keywords/KW-1161. Accessed 25 Dec. 2019.

Viral Fusion

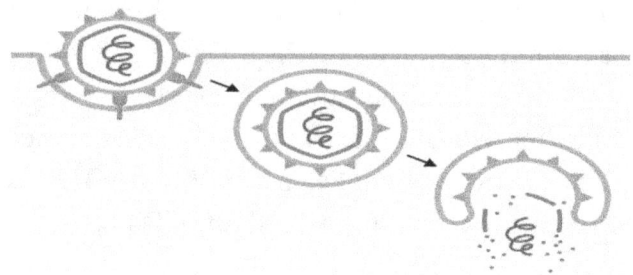

In the viral fusion, stage HIV injects proteins into the cellular fluids of the CD4 cell. In this stage, this is the fusion or joining of the host cell membranes to the outer part of HIV.[96] The fusion proteins triggered between viral and cellular membranes.[97] "All fusion proteins, in the fusion state, are active in a trimeric confirmation."[98] As a

---

[96] "Viral membrane fusion - ScienceDirect." https://www.sciencedirect.com/science/article/pii/S004268221500183X. Accessed 26 Dec. 2019.

[97] "Fusion of virus membrane with host cell membrane ...." https://viralzone.expasy.org/by_protein/987. Accessed 26 Dec. 2019.

[98] "Fusion of virus membrane with host cell membrane ...." https://viralzone.expasy.org/by_protein/987. Accessed 26 Dec. 2019.

part of the fusing, fusion pores develops, it creates a tunnel between the virus and the city for self.[99] It is through this tunnel that the HIV genetic material enters a healthy CD4 cell.[100]

The Encoding

HIV uses its material, RNA, for reproduction or making copies.[101] The protective coating or capsid surrounds the RNA strand must disassemble or took part.[102] In the encoding stage, the capsid organizers and contains viral RNA.[103] The viral RNA makes a delivery to the target cell

---

[99] "Viral membrane fusion. - NCBI - NIH." https://www.ncbi.nlm.nih.gov/pubmed/25866377. Accessed 26 Dec. 2019.

[100] "Viral membrane fusion. - NCBI - NIH." https://www.ncbi.nlm.nih.gov/pubmed/25866377. Accessed 26 Dec. 2019.

[101] "Living with HIV: A Patient's Guide, 2d ed.." https://books.google.com/books?id=Bo2SDgAAQBAJ&pg=PT48&lpg=PT48&dq=RNA+strand+must+be+disassembled&source=bl&ots=CVRwzS_H-o&sig=ACfU3U2jPG83vCnRKRUXBaa4BXBYgoBKFQ&hl=en. Accessed 26 Dec. 2019.

[102] "From DNA to RNA - Molecular Biology of the Cell - NCBI ...." https://www.ncbi.nlm.nih.gov/books/NBK26887/. Accessed 26 Dec. 2019.

[103] "The Information in DNA Determines Cellular Function via ...." https://www.nature.com/scitable/topicpage/the-information-in-dna-determines-cellular-function-6523228. Accessed 26 Dec. 2019.

or the CD4 cell[104] with two strands of RNA.[105]

The Reverse Transcription

Single-stranded HIV RNA converts to a double-stranded DNA[106] that helps enzyme reverse transcriptase helps in the reverse transcription process.[107]

The reverse transcriptase encodes from the genetic material of the retrovirus.[108] The reverse transcriptase uses

---

[104] "T7 RNA polymerase non-specifically transcribes and induces ...." 30 Apr. 2018, https://www.ncbi.nlm.nih.gov/pmc/articles/PMC6007251/. Accessed 26 Dec. 2019.

[105] "Living with HIV: A Patient's Guide, 2d ed.." https://books.google.com/books?id=Bo2SDgAAQBAJ&pg=PT48&lpg=PT48&dq=RNA+strand+must+be+disassembled&source=bl&ots=CVRwzS_H-o&sig=ACfU3U2jPG83vCnRKRUXBaa4BXBYgoBKFQ&hl=en. Accessed 26 Dec. 2019.

[106] "Reverse Transcription Basics | Thermo Fisher Scientific - US." https://www.thermofisher.com/us/en/home/life-science/cloning/cloning-learning-center/invitrogen-school-of-molecular-biology/rt-education/reverse-transcription-basics.html. Accessed 26 Dec. 2019.

[107] "Overview of Reverse Transcription - Retroviruses - NCBI ...." https://www.ncbi.nlm.nih.gov/books/NBK19424/. Accessed 26 Dec. 2019.

[108] "Overview of Reverse Transcription - Retroviruses - NCBI ...." https://www.ncbi.nlm.nih.gov/books/NBK19424/. Accessed 26 Dec.

proteins from the CD4 cell [109] and changes HIV RNA to HIV DNA. The DNA contains HIV genetic information required for HIV replication or making copies.[110]

Integration

Integrating HIV DNA directly into host DNA is a dire step in the HIV life cycle.[111] In the integration stage, the virus goes inside the nucleus and releases an enzyme known as retroviral integrase.[112] This enzyme is responsible for a chemical reaction that takes place in the nucleus and can cause the transfer of viral DNA into the CD4 cells.[113] In

---

2019.

[109] "Reverse Transcription (cDNA Synthesis) | NEB." https://www.neb.com/applications/cloning-and-synthetic-biology/dna-preparation/reverse-transcription-cdna-synthesis. Accessed 26 Dec. 2019.

[110] "Reverse transcriptase | enzyme | Britannica." https://www.britannica.com/science/reverse-transcriptase. Accessed 26 Dec. 2019.

[111] "HIV DNA Integration - NCBI." https://www.ncbi.nlm.nih.gov/pmc/articles/PMC3385939/. Accessed 26 Dec. 2019.

[112] "Integration | Definition | AIDSinfo." https://aidsinfo.nih.gov/understanding-hiv-aids/glossary/381/integration. Accessed 26 Dec. 2019.

[113] "HIV DNA Integration." 8 May. 2012, http://perspectivesinmedicine.cshlp.org/content/2/7/a006890.abstract. Accessed 26 Dec. 2019.

this stage, HIV inserts the enzyme integrase into the CD4 cell's DNA.[114]

Understanding the integration process will offer a background for attaining viewpoint into multiple potential sites of therapeutic involvement for HIV infection and AIDS.[115] HIV's enzyme inserted in the DNA of its genome diametrically into host cell DNA is the "integrase stage."[116] HIV-1 integrase catalyzes the "cut-and-paste" action of cutting the DNA and linking the proviral genome towards the cut ends.[117]

Viral Latency

In the viral latency stage, this stage is the waiting period

---

[114] "Integration of HIV in the Human Genome: Which Sites Are ...." 24 Apr. 2016, https://www.hindawi.com/journals/ijg/2016/2168590/. Accessed 26 Dec. 2019.

[115] "The role of integration and clonal expansion in HIV infection ...." 23 Oct. 2018, https://retrovirology.biomedcentral.com/articles/10.1186/s12977-018-0448-8. Accessed 26 Dec. 2019.

[116] "The role of integration and clonal expansion in HIV infection ...." 23 Oct. 2018, https://retrovirology.biomedcentral.com/articles/10.1186/s12977-018-0448-8. Accessed 26 Dec. 2019.

[117] "Integration of HIV in the Human Genome: Which Sites Are ...." 24 Apr. 2016, https://www.hindawi.com/journals/ijg/2016/2168590/. Accessed 26 Dec. 2019.

or the incubation period. When a virus exists in the body, but occurs in a relaxing (inactive) state without ever producing more viruses.[118] A latent viral infection rarely causes any apparent symptoms and could last a long period before becoming dynamic and resulting in symptoms.[119] HIV can manage viral latency, as seen in the reservoirs of latent HIV-infected cells that persist within a person's body despite antiretroviral therapy (ART).[120] When the viral DNA goes through the integration stage, that virus is latent.[121] Some call the virus, provirus. The virus waits to and then becomes active.[122] The provirus in this stage causes the cells to make proteins and components of

---

[118] "Viral Latency | Definition | AIDSinfo."
https://aidsinfo.nih.gov/understanding-hiv-aids/glossary/408/viral-latency. Accessed 26 Dec. 2019.

[119] "Viral Latency | Definition | AIDSinfo."
https://aidsinfo.nih.gov/understanding-hiv-aids/glossary/408/viral-latency. Accessed 26 Dec. 2019.

[120] "Viral latency and its regulation: lessons from the - NCBI."
https://www.ncbi.nlm.nih.gov/pmc/articles/PMC2914632/.
Accessed 26 Dec. 2019.

[121] "Viral latency ~ ViralZone page."
https://viralzone.expasy.org/by_protein/3970. Accessed 26 Dec. 2019.

[122] "Viral latency - UniProt."
https://www.uniprot.org/keywords/KW-1251. Accessed 26 Dec. 2019.

Final Assembly

In the last assembly stage of HIV, the viral protein cut into pieces and assemble into new-viruses.[124] It accompanies the cleavage or the cutting with help from an enzyme known as protease.[125] In the last assembly stage, it cut the protein into smaller particles. These proteins are from the segment form of HIV proteins.[126] The new HIV formed protein and viral is in a move to the surface of the CD4 cells.[127] This process assembles into what we know as an immature (non-infectious) copy of HIV.[128]

---

[123] "Herpes Simplex Virus Latency: The DNA Repair-Centered ...." 16 Jan. 2017, https://www.hindawi.com/journals/av/2017/7028194/. Accessed 26 Dec. 2019.

[124] "Assembly | Definition | AIDSinfo." https://aidsinfo.nih.gov/understanding-hiv-aids/glossary/4593/assembly. Accessed 26 Dec. 2019.

[125] "The HIV Life Cycle | Understanding HIV/AIDS | AIDSinfo." 1 Jul. 2019, https://aidsinfo.nih.gov/understanding-hiv-aids/fact-sheets/19/73/the-hiv-life-cycle. Accessed 26 Dec. 2019.

[126] "HIV-1 Assembly, Budding, and Maturation - NCBI - NIH." https://www.ncbi.nlm.nih.gov/pmc/articles/PMC3385941/. Accessed 26 Dec. 2019.

[127] "The Structural Biology of HIV Assembly - NCBI - NIH." https://www.ncbi.nlm.nih.gov/pmc/articles/PMC2819415/. Accessed 26 Dec. 2019.

[128] "HIV-1 assembly in macrophages | Retrovirology | Full Text." 7

Budding or Maturation

The budding or maturation stage of HIV is the last stage of the HIV life cycle.[129] The new-created HIV, complete with viral genetic material along with a new outer coat made from the cell membrane of the host CD4 or helper cell.[130]

The new-formed virus pinches off or takes part in the host cell and enters the body's circulation.[131] After a period of maturation, and HIV forms into a new-created HIV cell, which takes aggressive action against another CD4 cell and starts the process over again.[132]

Apr. 2010, https://retrovirology.biomedcentral.com/articles/10.1186/1742-4690-7-29. Accessed 26 Dec. 2019.

[129] "HIV maturation: early draft – Science of HIV." http://scienceofhiv.org/wp/?portfolio=hiv-maturation-early-draft. Accessed 26 Dec. 2019.

[130] "HIV-1 Assembly, Budding, and Maturation - NCBI - NIH." https://www.ncbi.nlm.nih.gov/pmc/articles/PMC3385941/. Accessed 26 Dec. 2019.

[131] "Budding | Definition | AIDSinfo." https://aidsinfo.nih.gov/understanding-hiv-aids/glossary/814/budding. Accessed 26 Dec. 2019.

[132] "HIV-1 assembly, budding, and maturation. - NCBI - NIH." https://www.ncbi.nlm.nih.gov/pubmed/22762019. Accessed 26 Dec. 2019.

Chapter 3 Adherence to taking Medications

Adherence

When talking about adherence, there are several components that the patient needs to do, or the peer educator should discuss? Such as treatment adherence include starting HIV treatment and keeping all their medical appointments and taking medications every day as prescribed by the medical professional. [133] For people with HIV treatment, the key is staying healthy. It is best to see a health care provider as soon as possible after testing positive for HIV.[134] Once the patient is in medical care, people with HIV should start taking HIV medication as soon as possible. Because HIV requires a long-life treatment, it is essential for people with HIV to visit their healthcare provider regularly.[135]

---

[133] "The challenge of patient adherence - NCBI." https://www.ncbi.nlm.nih.gov/pmc/articles/PMC1661624/. Accessed 26 Dec. 2019.

[134] "HIV Treatment Adherence | Understanding HIV/AIDS | AIDSinfo." 18 Feb. 2019, https://aidsinfo.nih.gov/understanding-hiv-aids/fact-sheets/21/54/hiv-treatment-adherence. Accessed 26 Dec. 2019.

[135] "The importance of treatment adherence in HIV. - NCBI." https://www.ncbi.nlm.nih.gov/pubmed/24495293. Accessed 26

WHAT PEER EDUCATORS IN HIV EDUCATION AND PATIENTS SHOULD KNOW

What is HIV treatment, adherence?

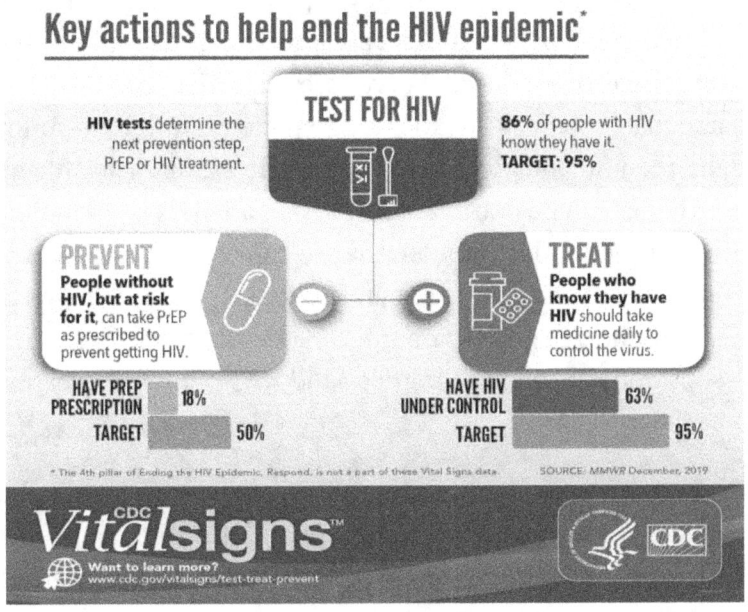

Adherent means to stick firmly on here to something. For people with HIV, treatment adherence includes several things. Quality healthcare outcomes will depend upon the patient adherence to recommended treatment regimens.[136]

Dec. 2019.

[136] "HIV Treatment Adherence | Understanding HIV/AIDS | AIDSinfo." 18 Feb. 2019, https://aidsinfo.nih.gov/understanding-hiv-aids/fact-sheets/21/54/hiv-treatment-adherence. Accessed 26 Dec.

Patient, not adherence can be a pervasive threat to their health and their well-being and carry a substantial economic burden.

For most medical conditions, correct diagnosis and effective medical treatment are essential to patient survival and quality of life. There are significant barriers to adequate medical treatment. The patient's failure to follow the recommendation of his or her physician or healthcare provider can be detrimental.[137] The patient is nonadherent, sometimes called noncompliance can take many forms.[138] Sometimes the patient misunderstands the advice given by a healthcare professional. [139]Non-adherents care is a substantial economic burden, and it is putting the patient at risk.

None inherent compromise this patient's outcomes, but this is most apparent when the patient does not take the

---

2019.

[137] "HIV Treatment Adherence | Understanding HIV/AIDS | AIDSinfo." 18 Feb. 2019, https://aidsinfo.nih.gov/understanding-hiv-aids/fact-sheets/21/54/hiv-treatment-adherence. Accessed 26 Dec. 2019.

[138] "Improving the Adherence to Antiretroviral Therapy, a Difficult ...." https://www.ncbi.nlm.nih.gov/pmc/articles/PMC5703840/. Accessed 26 Dec. 2019.

[139] "Improving the Adherence to Antiretroviral Therapy, a Difficult ...." https://www.ncbi.nlm.nih.gov/pmc/articles/PMC5703840/. Accessed 26 Dec. 2019.

medication.[140] A patient suffering any disease adherence jeopardizes their survival.[141] Adherence to the medication for controlling the disease is essential in preventing an opportunistic infection.

Interpersonal Relationship Role

The key to success is the interpersonal relationship. Interpersonal relationships, with both the peer educator and the patient, play a role in the outcomes.

The patient who feels that their peer educator communicates well with them and actively encourages them to help the patient take charge of their care.[142] That means successful communication between the peers promotes greater patient satisfaction intern fosters a top level of adherence.[143]

---

[140] "Adherence | Limitations to Treatment Safety and Efficacy ...." 17 Oct. 2017, https://aidsinfo.nih.gov/guidelines/html/1/adult-and-adolescent-arv/30/adherence. Accessed 26 Dec. 2019.

[141] "HIV Treatment Adherence - POZ." https://www.poz.com/basics/hiv-basics/hiv-treatment-adherence. Accessed 26 Dec. 2019.

[142] "Different Types of Interpersonal Relationships." https://www.managementstudyguide.com/types-of-interpersonal-relationships.htm. Accessed 26 Dec. 2019.

[143] "How to Maintain Strong Interpersonal Relationships - Lifehack." 20 Aug. 2019, https://www.lifehack.org/842962/interpersonal-relationship. Accessed 26 Dec. 2019.

The more patients know, the more likely the patient will be interested in managing their disease and stick to taking their medications regime. Another critical factor that can improve patient-related medication adherence, the peer needs to be active with patient and treatment decisions when possible. A straightforward way to improve a patient's adherence is to ask what time a day they preferred to take their medications, or when do they take their medications. One patient might be more likely to adhere to his or her medications if they were taking them in the evening, whereas another morning.

Other factors are beneficial in adherence, and this would include starting HIV treatment, keeping all medical appointments, and taking HIV medicines every day and as prescribed.[144] For people with HIV, treatment adherence, as stated earlier, is staying healthy.[145]

Why is medication adherence significant to the patient?

Taking HIV medications every day prevents HIV from

---

[144] "Interpersonal relationship - ScienceDaily."
https://www.sciencedaily.com/terms/interpersonal_relationship.htm. Accessed 26 Dec. 2019.

[145] "Interpersonal Relationships: How to Maintain Them - Healthline." 22 Oct. 2018,
https://www.healthline.com/health/interpersonal-relationships. Accessed 26 Dec. 2019.

multiplying in an individual's body.[146] Adherence reduces the risk of HIV.[147] Being nonadherent will cause the virus to mutate and produce drug resistance to HIV. Mutation happens, and permanent change in the genetic material of a cell or microorganism takes place.[148] A nonadherent patient who has a mutation can harm themselves and the other person because the microorganisms replicate.[149] HIV mutations trigger the virus to become resilient to specific antiretroviral drugs.[150]

Why did the patient forget to take the medication?

There is a variance between an infrequently missed dose and habitually overlooking on a daily or weekly basis. The

---

[146] "The Basics of HIV Prevention | Understanding HIV/AIDS ...." 29 Apr. 2019, https://aidsinfo.nih.gov/understanding-hiv-aids/fact-sheets/20/48/the-basics-of-hiv-prevention. Accessed 26 Dec. 2019.

[147] "HIV prevention | UNAIDS."
https://www.unaids.org/en/topic/prevention. Accessed 26 Dec. 2019.

[148] "The Genetic Mutation Behind the Only Apparent Cure for HIV ...." 14 Mar. 2019, https://www.thebodypro.com/article/genetic-mutation-behind-hiv-cure. Accessed 26 Dec. 2019.

[149] "Genetic Mutation that Prevents HIV Infection Tied to Earlier ...." 3 Jun. 2019, https://www.the-scientist.com/news-opinion/genetic-mutation-that-prevents-hiv-infection-tied-to-earlier-death-65960. Accessed 26 Dec. 2019.

[150] "The Genetic Mutation Behind the Only Apparent Cure for HIV ...." 14 Mar. 2019, https://www.thebodypro.com/article/genetic-mutation-behind-hiv-cure. Accessed 26 Dec. 2019.

patient needs to be strict when adherent to their medication. The peer educator could suggest a timer for the patient, record the time they take the medication in a logbook, calendar, or planner.[151] The peer could also suggest taking their medication based on their favorite show on television. The patient needs a regimen that they can follow every day; this includes both doing the weekends and in different situations involved in their life. Skipping HIV medications causes HIV to multiply many times in the body.[152] This multiplication of HIV in the bloodstream increases the risk of drug resistance and HIV treatment failure.[153]

Asking questions concerning medications

The next step and helping the patient to be adhering to the medication is that the peer needs to ask questions. By asking the questions to peer, can accurately assess which medications the patients are taking and how they are taking these medications.[154] The peer educator may ask the

---

[151] "Effectiveness of Peer Education Interventions for HIV - NCBI." https://www.ncbi.nlm.nih.gov/pmc/articles/PMC3927325/. Accessed 26 Dec. 2019.

[152] "HIV Drug Resistance Database." https://hivdb.stanford.edu/. Accessed 26 Dec. 2019.

[153] "HIV Resistant Mutation | Viruses101 | Learn Science at Scitable." 6 Oct. 2013, https://www.nature.com/scitable/blog/viruses101/hiv_resistant_mutation. Accessed 26 Dec. 2019.

[154] "Peer education in HIV prevention: an evaluation in schools." 23

patient twice to list their medications. Listing medications does not tell the peer educator whether the patient is taking their medications. If the peer educator assumes that the patient is taking the medication, this may not be true.[155] The peer educator assesses the patient's medication by asking several direct questions in a very non-judgmental manner.[156]

Questions:

1. I know that it must be tough for you to take your medication.
2. How often do you miss taking your medications?
3. Of the medications the doctor prescribed to you, which ones are you taking?
4. In what manner often do you not take medication X? The peer educator should address each medication individually.

Jan. 2006, https://www.ncbi.nlm.nih.gov/pubmed/16431871. Accessed 26 Dec. 2019.

[155] "Effects of peer education intervention on HIV/AIDS related ...." 7 Sep. 2015, https://www.ncbi.nlm.nih.gov/pmc/articles/PMC4562206/. Accessed 26 Dec. 2019.

[156] "Effectiveness of peer education interventions for HIV ...." 28 May. 2012, https://academic.oup.com/her/article/27/5/904/579723. Accessed 26 Dec. 2019.

5. When did you last take the medication X that the doctor prescribed?
6. Have you noticed any side effects from your medications?

These are questions to get the conversation started.

Chapter 4 PreP as Prevention

Using PrEP as Prevention

Pre-exposure prophylaxis is a new HIV prevention approach where HIV-negative individuals use anti-HIV medication to lessen their risk of exposure to the virus.[157] It is a supplementary tool for persons to consider in HIV prevention.[158]

The pre- means before.[159] Exposure means coming into contact with HIV.[160] Prophylaxis means treat to prevent an

---

[157] "PrEP | HIV Basics | HIV/AIDS | CDC." https://www.cdc.gov/hiv/basics/prep.html. Accessed 27 Dec. 2019.

[158] "Pre-Exposure Prophylaxis (PrEP) | HIV Risk and Prevention ...." https://www.cdc.gov/hiv/risk/prep/index.html. Accessed 27 Dec. 2019.

[159] "PrEP | HIV Basics | HIV/AIDS | CDC." https://www.cdc.gov/hiv/basics/prep.html. Accessed 27 Dec. 2019.

[160] "Pre-Exposure Prophylaxis (PrEP) | HIV Risk and Prevention ...." https://www.cdc.gov/hiv/risk/prep/index.html. Accessed 27 Dec. 2019.

infection from happening.[161]

Prophylaxis is an HIV prevention strategy where HIV-negative individuals take the anti-HIV medication before coming in contact with HIV.[162] The purpose of taking this medication is to reduce the risk of becoming infected.[163] The medication works to prevent HIV from establishing infection inside the person's body.[164]

PrEP diminishes the risk of HIV infection through sex for a gay and bisexual man, transgender women, and heterosexual men and women, and among people who inject drugs.[165] It does not guard them against sexually transmitted infections or pregnancy. It is not a cure for

---

[161] "Pre-Exposure Prophylaxis (PrEP) | HIV Risk and Prevention ...." https://www.cdc.gov/hiv/risk/prep/index.html. Accessed 27 Dec. 2019.

[162] "Pre-Exposure Prophylaxis (PrEP) | HIV Risk and Prevention ...." https://www.cdc.gov/hiv/risk/prep/index.html. Accessed 27 Dec. 2019.

[163] "Pre-Exposure Prophylaxis (PrEP) | HIV Risk and Prevention ...." https://www.cdc.gov/hiv/risk/prep/index.html. Accessed 27 Dec. 2019.

[164] "Pre-Exposure Prophylaxis (PrEP) | HIV Risk and Prevention ...." https://www.cdc.gov/hiv/risk/prep/index.html. Accessed 27 Dec. 2019.

[165] "The Basics - PrEP." https://prepfacts.org/prep/the-basics/. Accessed 27 Dec. 2019.

HIV.[166]

Differences between prep and pep

Post means after. Exposure means coming into contact with HIV. Prophylaxis means treatment to prevent HIV infection from happening.[167] Post-exposure prophylaxis is an HIV prevention strategy with HIV-negative individuals.[168] The individual takes HIV medications after coming in contact with HIV to lessen their possibility of infection.[169] PEP is a month-long course of prescriptions, and one must within 72 hours after exposure to an individual who may be HIV positive.[170]

---

[166] "The Basics - PrEP." https://prepfacts.org/prep/the-basics/. Accessed 27 Dec. 2019.

[167] "What is pre-exposure prophylaxis (PrEP)? | Avert." 26 Sep. 2019, https://www.avert.org/hiv-transmission-prevention/prep. Accessed 27 Dec. 2019.

[168] "Pre-exposure prophylaxis (PrEP) for HIV prevention | Avert." 3 Oct. 2019, https://www.avert.org/professionals/hiv-programming/prevention/pre-exposure-prophylaxis. Accessed 27 Dec. 2019.

[169] "Pre-Exposure Prophylaxis | HIV.gov." 3 Dec. 2019, https://www.hiv.gov/hiv-basics/hiv-prevention/using-hiv-medication-to-reduce-risk/pre-exposure-prophylaxis. Accessed 27 Dec. 2019.

[170] "Pre-Exposure Prophylaxis | HIV.gov." 3 Dec. 2019, https://www.hiv.gov/hiv-basics/hiv-prevention/using-hiv-medication-to-reduce-risk/pre-exposure-prophylaxis. Accessed 27

Chapter 5 U=U

U=U in HIV care

Undetectable equals on transmittable is a recent phenomenon in HIV care. Did U=U campaign recognizes the clear scientific evidence showing that a person with HIV who has a repressed viral load will not transfer HIV to their sexual partners? Combine data from 2008 to 2016 showed that there was zero link HIV transmission after over 100,000 condomless sex acts with them both heterosexual and male to male serodiscordant couples where the partners living with HIV had an undetectable viral load.

There was a study that researchers did to prove the evidence that undetectable equals transmittable.[171] A randomized clinical trial and observational cohort studies tested the effects of viral suppression and preventing HIV transmission.[172] The studies followed male couples in which one partner was HIV positive and the other HIV negative.[173] During the studies, there were zero link HIV

Dec. 2019.

[171] "Undetectable = Untransmittable (U=U) - Minnesota Dept. of ...." https://www.health.state.mn.us/diseases/hiv/prevention/uu/index.html. Accessed 27 Dec. 2019.

[172] "Undetectable = Untransmittable (U=U) - Minnesota Dept. of ...." https://www.health.state.mn.us/diseases/hiv/prevention/uu/index.html. Accessed 27 Dec. 2019.

[173] "Undetectable = Untransmittable (U=U) - Minnesota Dept. of ...."

transmission documented when the HIV positive receiving antiretroviral therapy.[174] That means there were fewer than 200 copies per milliliter and the individual's blood system.[175] There were over 1800 couples year of follow-up in the observational cohort starting male couples.[176] The couples had anal sex without condoms over 34,000 times, and heterosexual couples had vaginal or anal sex without condoms over 36,000 times with zero link to HIV transmission.[177]

What does suppression mean when talking about U=U?

The advance of antiretroviral drugs to treat HIV has turned wet ones and almost always fatal infection into a

---

https://www.health.state.mn.us/diseases/hiv/prevention/uu/index.html. Accessed 27 Dec. 2019.

[174] "Prevention Access Campaign: U=U | United States." https://www.preventionaccess.org/. Accessed 27 Dec. 2019.

[175] "Undetectable = Untransmittable (U=U) - Minnesota Dept. of ...." https://www.health.state.mn.us/diseases/hiv/prevention/uu/index.html. Accessed 27 Dec. 2019.

[176] "Prevention Access Campaign: U=U | United States." https://www.preventionaccess.org/. Accessed 27 Dec. 2019.

[177] "Undetectable = Untransmittable (U=U) - Minnesota Dept. of ...." https://www.health.state.mn.us/diseases/hiv/prevention/uu/index.html. Accessed 27 Dec. 2019.

manageable chronic disease. Daily antiretroviral therapy can decrease the quantity of HIV in the blood two levels undetectable with standard tests. Staying on the treatment is crucial to keep the virus suppressed research has documented and showed that achieving and maintaining undetectable viral load not only preserve the health of the person living with HIV but prevent sexual transmission of the virus to an HIV-negative partner.

Antiretroviral therapy represses HIV from making duplicates of itself. When a person living with HIV begins and antiretroviral treatment regimen, their viral load drops. For almost everyone who starts taking the HIV medication daily as prescribed, viral loads will become undetectable in six months or fewer — continuing to take HIV medication as directed is imperative to stay on detectable.

Taking antiretroviral therapy every day as prescribed to suppress HIV levels leads to an undetectable status. A person who has undetectable viral load if they remain undetectable for at least six months following their first undetectable test results. It is essential to continue taking the medication every day as directed to maintain an on detectable viral load.

Even when a viral load is barely discernible, HIV is still present in the human body. The virus lies latent inside an insignificant number of cells in the body identified as viral reservoirs. When therapy stops by missing doses, taking a treatment holiday, or stopping treatment, the virus emerges and multiplies, becoming detectable in the blood again. This new reducing virus is infectious. It is critical to take every pill every day as instructed to attain and sustain a and undetectable status.

References

10 Things Everyone Should Understand About HIV And AIDS. 28 Oct. 2016, https://www.self.com/story/facts-about-hiv-and-aids. Accessed 25 Dec. 2019.

A Timeline of HIV and AIDS | HIV.gov. https://www.hiv.gov/hiv-basics/overview/history/hiv-and-aids-timeline. Accessed 27 Dec. 2019.

Adherence | Limitations to Treatment Safety and Efficacy. 17 Oct. 2017, https://aidsinfo.nih.gov/guidelines/html/1/adult-and-adolescent-arv/30/adherence. Accessed 26 Dec. 2019.

AIDS Timeline. http://www.factlv.org/timeline.htm. Accessed 27 Dec. 2019.

Antiretroviral Therapy for HIV Infection: Overview, FDA. 18 Apr. 2019, https://emedicine.medscape.com/article/1533218-overview. Accessed 25 Dec. 2019.

ART access-related barriers faced by HIV-positive persons. 7 Dec. 2016, https://www.ncbi.nlm.nih.gov/pmc/articles/PMC5142337/. Accessed 27 Dec. 2019.

Assembly | Definition | AIDSinfo. https://aidsinfo.nih.gov/understanding-hiv-aids/glossary/4593/assembly. Accessed 26 Dec. 2019.

Beyond the Cut Hunter: A Historical Epidemiology of HIV. https://www.ncbi.nlm.nih.gov/pubmed/27718030. Accessed 25 Dec. 2019.

Beyond the Cut Hunter: A Historical Epidemiology of HIV. https://www.ncbi.nlm.nih.gov/pubmed/27718030. Accessed 25 Dec. 2019.

Budding | Definition | AIDSinfo. https://aidsinfo.nih.gov/understanding-hiv-aids/glossary/814/budding. Accessed 26 Dec. 2019.

CD4 cell counts | aidsmap. 31 May. 2017, https://www.aidsmap.com/about-hiv/cd4-cell-counts. Accessed 25 Dec. 2019.

CD4 Count, HIV, and AIDS: Test and Results, What They Mean. 23 Jun. 2019, https://www.webmd.com/hiv-aids/cd4-count-what-does-it-mean. Accessed 25 Dec. 2019.

Different Types of Interpersonal Relationships.https://www.managementstudyguide.com/types-of-interpersonal-relationships.htm. Accessed 26 Dec. 2019.

Dissecting How CD4 T Cells Are Lost During HIV Infection. https://www.ncbi.nlm.nih.gov/pmc/articles/PMC4835240/. Accessed 26 Dec. 2019.

DNA (Deoxyribonucleic Acid) | Talking Glossary of

Genetic https://www.genome.gov/genetics-glossary/Deoxyribonucleic-Acid. Accessed 25 Dec. 2019.

Effectiveness of Peer Education Interventions for HIV - NCBI. https://www.ncbi.nlm.nih.gov/pmc/articles/PMC3927325/. Accessed 26 Dec. 2019.

Effects of a peer education intervention on HIV/AIDS related. 7 Sep. 2015, https://www.ncbi.nlm.nih.gov/pmc/articles/PMC4562206/. Accessed 26 Dec. 2019.

From DNA to RNA - Molecular Biology of the Cell – NCBI. https://www.ncbi.nlm.nih.gov/books/NBK26887/. Accessed 26 Dec. 2019.

Fusion of virus membrane with host cell membrane .... https://viralzone.expasy.org/by_protein/987. Accessed 26 Dec. 2019.

Genetic Mutation that Prevents HIV Infection Tied to Earlier .... 3 Jun. 2019, https://www.the-scientist.com/news-opinion/genetic-mutation-that-prevents-hiv-infection-tied-to-earlier-death-65960. Accessed 26 Dec. 2019.

Here's Why the First Cure for HIV Could Emerge from .... 5 Nov. 2019, https://biobuzz.io/heres-why-the-first-cure-for-hiv-could-emerge-from-maryland/. Accessed 27

Dec. 2019.

Herpes Simplex Virus Latency: The DNA Repair-Centered .... 16 Jan. 2017, https://www.hindawi.com/journals/av/2017/7028194/. Accessed 26 Dec. 2019.

History of HIV and AIDS overview | Avert. https://www.avert.org/professionals/history-hiv-aids/overview. Accessed 27 Dec. 2019.

HIV DNA Integration - NCBI. https://www.ncbi.nlm.nih.gov/pmc/articles/PMC3385939/. Accessed 26 Dec. 2019.

HIV DNA Integration. 8 May. 2012, http://perspectivesinmedicine.cshlp.org/content/2/7/a006890.abstract. Accessed 26 Dec. 2019.

HIV Drug Resistance Database. https://hivdb.stanford.edu/. Accessed 26 Dec. 2019.

HIV maturation: early draft – Science of HIV. http://scienceofhiv.org/wp/?portfolio=hiv-maturation-early-draft. Accessed 26 Dec. 2019.

HIV Medications: Combinations, Antiretrovirals, HAART, & More. 20 Oct. 2019, https://www.webmd.com/hiv-aids/hiv-medications. Accessed 27 Dec. 2019.

HIV Medications: NRTIs, Protease Inhibitors, and Much

More. https://www.healthline.com/health/hiv-aids/medications-list. Accessed 27 Dec. 2019.

HIV Medications: NRTIs, Protease Inhibitors, and Much More. https://www.healthline.com/health/hiv-aids/medications-list. Accessed 27 Dec. 2019.

HIV Medicines and Side Effects | Understanding HIV/AIDS .... 24 Oct. 2019, https://aidsinfo.nih.gov/understanding-hiv-aids/fact-sheets/22/63/hiv-medicines-and-side-effects. Accessed 27 Dec. 2019.

HIV prevention | UNAIDS. https://www.unaids.org/en/topic/prevention. Accessed 26 Dec. 2019.

HIV Resistant Mutation | Viruses101 | Learn Science at Scitable. 6 Oct. 2013, https://www.nature.com/scitable/blog/viruses101/hiv_resistant_mutation. Accessed 26 Dec. 2019.

HIV Treatment Adherence - POZ. https://www.poz.com/basics/hiv-basics/hiv-treatment-adherence. Accessed 26 Dec. 2019.

HIV Treatment Adherence | Understanding HIV/AIDS | AIDSinfo. 18 Feb. 2019, https://aidsinfo.nih.gov/understanding-hiv-aids/fact-sheets/21/54/hiv-treatment-adherence. Accessed 26 Dec. 2019.

HIV Treatment Adherence | Understanding HIV/AIDS | AIDSinfo. 18 Feb. 2019, https://aidsinfo.nih.gov/understanding-hiv-aids/fact-sheets/21/54/hiv-treatment-adherence. Accessed 26 Dec. 2019.

HIV Treatment Adherence | Understanding HIV/AIDS | AIDSinfo. 18 Feb. 2019, https://aidsinfo.nih.gov/understanding-hiv-aids/fact-sheets/21/54/hiv-treatment-adherence. Accessed 26 Dec. 2019.

HIV virologic response better with single-tablet once daily .... 4 Dec. 2018, https://www.ncbi.nlm.nih.gov/pmc/articles/PMC6295695/. Accessed 27 Dec. 2019.

HIV: Antiretroviral Therapy (ART) - Types, Brand Names, How. 22 Oct. 2019, https://www.webmd.com/hiv-aids/aids-hiv-medication. Accessed 27 Dec. 2019.

HIV: from a devastating epidemic to a manageable ... - WHO. https://www.who.int/publications/10-year-review/hiv/en/. Accessed 25 Dec. 2019.

HIV-1 assembly in macrophages | Retrovirology | Full Text. 7 Apr. 2010, https://retrovirology.biomedcentral.com/articles/10.1186/1742-4690-7-29. Accessed 26 Dec. 2019.

HIV-1 Assembly, Budding, and Maturation - NCBI - NIH. https://www.ncbi.nlm.nih.gov/pmc/articles/PMC3385941/. Accessed 26 Dec. 2019.

HIV-1 assembly, budding, and maturation. - NCBI - NIH. https://www.ncbi.nlm.nih.gov/pubmed/22762019. Accessed 26 Dec. 2019.

How HIV became a treatable, chronic disease. 2 Dec. 2015, http://theconversation.com/how-hiv-became-a-treatable-chronic-disease-51238. Accessed 25 Dec. 2019.

How HIV Infects a Cell | International Partnership For .... https://www.ipmglobal.org/how-hiv-infects-cell. Accessed 27 Dec. 2019.

How to Maintain Strong Interpersonal Relationships - Lifehack. 20 Aug. 2019, https://www.lifehack.org/842962/interpersonal-relationship. Accessed 26 Dec. 2019.

Improving the Adherence to Antiretroviral Therapy, a Difficult .... https://www.ncbi.nlm.nih.gov/pmc/articles/PMC5703840/. Accessed 26 Dec. 2019.

Integration | Definition | AIDSinfo. https://aidsinfo.nih.gov/understanding-hiv-aids/glossary/381/integration. Accessed 26 Dec. 2019.

Integration of HIV in the Human Genome: Which Sites

Are .... 24 Apr. 2016, https://www.hindawi.com/journals/ijg/2016/2168590/. Accessed 26 Dec. 2019.

Interpersonal relationship - ScienceDaily. https://www.sciencedaily.com/terms/interpersonal_relationship.htm. Accessed 26 Dec. 2019.

Interpersonal Relationships: How to Maintain Them - Healthline. 22 Oct. 2018, https://www.healthline.com/health/interpersonal-relationships. Accessed 26 Dec. 2019.

Just Diagnosed: Next Steps After Testing Positive for HIV. 18 Jan. 2019, https://aidsinfo.nih.gov/understanding-hiv-aids/fact-sheets/21/65/just-diagnosed--next-steps-after-testing-positive-for-hiv. Accessed 25 Dec. 2019.

Life Cycle | Definition | AIDSinfo. https://aidsinfo.nih.gov/understanding-hiv-aids/glossary/1596/life-cycle. Accessed 25 Dec. 2019.

Living with HIV: A Patient's Guide, 2d ed.. https://books.google.com/books?id=Bo2SDgAAQBAJ&pg=PT48&lpg=PT48&dq=RNA+strand+must+be+disassembled&source=bl&ots=CVRwzS_H-o&sig=ACfU3U2jPG83vCnRKRUXBaa4BXBYgoBKFQ&hl=en. Accessed 26 Dec. 2019.

Living with HIV: What is it really like? - Medical News

Today. 13 Dec. 2018, https://www.medicalnewstoday.com/articles/323981.php. Accessed 25 Dec. 2019.

Man the Hunter' theory is debunked in new book | The Source. 18 Feb. 2006, https://source.wustl.edu/2006/02/man-the-hunter-theory-is-debunked-in-new-book/. Accessed 25 Dec. 2019.

Management of HIV/AIDS - Wikipedia. https://en.wikipedia.org/wiki/Management_of_HIV/AIDS. Accessed 27 Dec. 2019.

Opportunistic Infections and AIDS-Related Cancers - HIV InSite. 14 Sep. 2011, http://hivinsite.ucsf.edu/insite?page=pb-diag-04-00. Accessed 26 Dec. 2019.

Origin of HIV & AIDS | Avert. https://www.avert.org/professionals/history-hiv-aids/origin. Accessed 25 Dec. 2019.

Origin of HIV & AIDS | Avert. https://www.avert.org/professionals/history-hiv-aids/origin. Accessed 25 Dec. 2019.

Origins of HIV and the AIDS Pandemic - NCBI. https://www.ncbi.nlm.nih.gov/pmc/articles/PMC3234451/. Accessed 26 Dec. 2019.

Overview of Reverse Transcription - Retroviruses - NCBI. https://www.ncbi.nlm.nih.gov/books/NBK19424/.

Accessed 26 Dec. 2019.

Peer education in HIV prevention: an evaluation in schools. 23 Jan. 2006, https://www.ncbi.nlm.nih.gov/pubmed/16431871. Accessed 26 Dec. 2019.

Pre-Exposure Prophylaxis | HIV.gov. 3 Dec. 2019, https://www.hiv.gov/hiv-basics/hiv-prevention/using-hiv-medication-to-reduce-risk/pre-exposure-prophylaxis. Accessed 27 Dec. 2019.

PrEP | HIV Basics | HIV/AIDS | CDC. https://www.cdc.gov/hiv/basics/prep.html. Accessed 27 Dec. 2019.

Prevention Access Campaign: U=U | United States. https://www.preventionaccess.org/. Accessed 27 Dec. 2019.

Prevention Access Campaign: U=U | United States. https://www.preventionaccess.org/. Accessed 27 Dec. 2019.

Reverse transcriptase | enzyme | Britannica. https://www.britannica.com/science/reverse-transcriptase. Accessed 26 Dec. 2019.

Reverse Transcription (cDNA Synthesis) | NEB. https://www.neb.com/applications/cloning-and-synthetic-biology/dna-preparation/reverse-transcription-cdna-synthesis. Accessed 26 Dec. 2019.

Reverse Transcription Basics | Thermo Fisher Scientific - U.S. https://www.thermofisher.com/us/en/home/life-science/cloning/cloning-learning-center/invitrogen-school-of-molecular-biology/rt-education/reverse-transcription-basics.html. Accessed 26 Dec. 2019.

RNA transport - Latest research and news | Nature. https://www.nature.com/subjects/rna-transport. Accessed 25 Dec. 2019.

RNA Transport and Local Control of Translation - NCBI. https://www.ncbi.nlm.nih.gov/pmc/articles/PMC1850961/. Accessed 25 Dec. 2019.

Simian Immunodeficiency Virus - an overview | ScienceDirect. https://www.sciencedirect.com/topics/medicine-and-dentistry/simian-immunodeficiency-virus. Accessed 25 Dec. 2019.

Simian Immunodeficiency Virus (SIV) | Definition | AIDSinfo. https://aidsinfo.nih.gov/understanding-hiv-aids/glossary/660/simian-immunodeficiency-virus. Accessed 25 Dec. 2019.

Simian Immunodeficiency Virus (SIV) | Definition | AIDSinfo. https://aidsinfo.nih.gov/understanding-hiv-aids/glossary/660/simian-immunodeficiency-virus. Accessed 25 Dec. 2019.

Simian Immunodeficiency Virus Infection of

Chimpanzees. https://jvi.asm.org/content/79/7/3891. Accessed 25 Dec. 2019.

Simian Immunodeficiency Virus Infection of Chimpanzees. https://jvi.asm.org/content/79/7/3891. Accessed 25 Dec. 2019.

Single-tablet regimen for HIV: Benefits and drug chart. 10 Dec. 2018, https://www.medicalnewstoday.com/articles/323942.php. Accessed 27 Dec. 2019.

Single-tablet regimens | aidsmap. 13 Jun. 2019, http://www.aidsmap.com/about-hiv/single-tablet-regimens. Accessed 27 Dec. 2019.

T7 RNA polymerase non-specifically transcribes and induces . 30 Apr. 2018, https://www.ncbi.nlm.nih.gov/pmc/articles/PMC6007251/. Accessed 26 Dec. 2019.

The Basics - PrEP. https://prepfacts.org/prep/the-basics/. Accessed 27 Dec. 2019.

The Basics of HIV Prevention | Understanding HIV/AIDS. 29 Apr. 2019, https://aidsinfo.nih.gov/understanding-hiv-aids/fact-sheets/20/48/the-basics-of-hiv-prevention. Accessed 26 Dec. 2019.

The challenge of patient adherence - NCBI. https://www.ncbi.nlm.nih.gov/pmc/articles/PMC1661624

/. Accessed 26 Dec. 2019.

The Genetic Mutation Behind the Only Apparent Cure for HIV . 14 Mar. 2019, https://www.thebodypro.com/article/genetic-mutation-behind-hiv-cure. Accessed 26 Dec. 2019.

The HIV Life Cycle | Understanding HIV/AIDS | AIDSinfo. 1 Jul. 2019, https://aidsinfo.nih.gov/understanding-hiv-aids/fact-sheets/19/73/the-hiv-life-cycle. Accessed 26 Dec. 2019.

The importance of treatment adherence in HIV. - NCBI. https://www.ncbi.nlm.nih.gov/pubmed/24495293. Accessed 26 Dec. 2019.

The Information in DNA Determines Cellular Function via. https://www.nature.com/scitable/topicpage/the-information-in-dna-determines-cellular-function-6523228. Accessed 26 Dec. 2019.

The role of integration and clonal expansion in HIV infection. 23 Oct. 2018, https://retrovirology.biomedcentral.com/articles/10.1186/s12977-018-0448-8. Accessed 26 Dec. 2019.

The role of integration and clonal expansion in HIV infection. 23 Oct. 2018, https://retrovirology.biomedcentral.com/articles/10.1186/s12977-018-0448-8. Accessed 26 Dec. 2019.

The Structural Biology of HIV Assembly - NCBI - NIH.

https://www.ncbi.nlm.nih.gov/pmc/articles/PMC2819415/. Accessed 26 Dec. 2019.

Thirty Years of HIV/AIDS: Snapshots of an Epidemic - amfAR. https://www.amfar.org/thirty-years-of-hiv/aids-snapshots-of-an-epidemic/. Accessed 27 Dec. 2019.

Undetectable = Untransmittable (U=U) - Minnesota Dept. of . https://www.health.state.mn.us/diseases/hiv/prevention/uu/index.html. Accessed 27 Dec. 2019.

Viral attachment to host cell - UniProt. https://www.uniprot.org/keywords/KW-1161. Accessed 25 Dec. 2019.

Viral Infection | Viral Infection Symptoms | MedlinePlus. https://medlineplus.gov/viralinfections.html. Accessed 25 Dec. 2019.

Viral latency - UniProt. https://www.uniprot.org/keywords/KW-1251. Accessed 26 Dec. 2019.

Viral Latency | Definition | AIDSinfo. https://aidsinfo.nih.gov/understanding-hiv-aids/glossary/408/viral-latency. Accessed 26 Dec. 2019.

Viral latency ~ ViralZone page. https://viralzone.expasy.org/by_protein/3970. Accessed

WHAT PEER EDUCATORS IN HIV EDUCATION AND PATIENTS SHOULD KNOW

26 Dec. 2019.

Viral latency and its regulation: lessons from the - NCBI. https://www.ncbi.nlm.nih.gov/pmc/articles/PMC2914632/. Accessed 26 Dec. 2019.

Virus Attachment - an overview | ScienceDirect Topics. https://www.sciencedirect.com/topics/medicine-and-dentistry/virus-attachment. Accessed 25 Dec. 2019.

Viruses: Structure, Function, and Uses - Molecular Cell. https://www.ncbi.nlm.nih.gov/books/NBK21523/. Accessed 25 Dec. 2019.

Viruses: Structure, Function, and Uses - Molecular Cell. https://www.ncbi.nlm.nih.gov/books/NBK21523/. Accessed 25 Dec. 2019.

What Are Viruses? | Live Science. 6 Jan. 2016, https://www.livescience.com/53272-what-is-a-virus.html. Accessed 25 Dec. 2019.

What is DNA? - Genetics Home Reference - NIH. 10 Dec. 2019, https://ghr.nlm.nih.gov/primer/basics/dna. Accessed 25 Dec. 2019.

What is pre-exposure prophylaxis (PrEP)? | Avert. 26 Sep. 2019, https://www.avert.org/hiv-transmission-prevention/prep. Accessed 27 Dec. 2019.

ABOUT THE AUTHOR

I have a B.S. degree from the University of Arkansas, Pine Bluff Arkansas, B.R.E. in Religious Education from Carver Baptist College and Seminary, Kansas City, Missouri, Masters of Art in History, Masters of Divinity, D. Min. with a focus on Global Health and Wellness from the Saint Paul School of Theology, Leawood, Kansas, Certification in Community Health Worker, Metropolitan Community College, Kansas City, Missouri Trinity College of the Bible and theology Seminary, Ph.D., in Counseling and Ethics, Alabama, received 75 doctoral hours in Organizational Leadership with a focus on Behavior Health from Grand Canyon University, Phoenix, Arizona. Served as a chaplain, adjunct professor, and medical educator.

www.ingramcontent.com/pod-product-compliance
Lightning Source LLC
Chambersburg PA
CBHW070456220526
45466CB00004B/1844